Bloo
Understa   ~~... To Eat~~
& Why You Should Eat
Foods Based On Your
Blood Type

Includes Blood Type Diet Foods
To Eat According To Your
Blood Type, and Recipes You'll
Love

Sara Clark

Table of Contents

Introduction

Chapter 1 - Good and bad foods based on blood type

Chapter 2 - Why and how are foods given blood type classifications?

Chapter 3: Who is it for?

Chapter 4 - A model blood type diet plan

Chapter 5 - Blood type diet and weight loss

Chapter 6 - Blood type diet recipes

Conclusion

Highly Recommended Diet Books:

SPECIAL BONUS

Introduction

Thank you for downloading the book, "Blood Type Diet Foods".

This book contains proven steps and strategies on how to create a health conscious dietary plan suitable for your specific blood type.

Living well, staying strong and having an admirable physique are everyone's dream. To achieve this dream, some people are willing to spend huge amount of money to get the perfect diet chart, undergo extreme physical exercises and even take pills that have many adverse effects on the body. People resort to these measures because they do not feel happy with their physical conditions. Blood type diet is a relatively new, and increasingly popular idea. This diet's popularity stems from it being easily adoptable, noticeably effective and completely safe.

The concept of blood type diet was first brought to light by the naturopath Dr. Peter J. D'Adamo in his book "Eat Right 4 Your Type". That book is the first of its kind in this particular field of nutrition. The doctor believes that one's ABO blood type classification is the primary determinant for a healthy individual diet, and that there are certain foods which are beneficial for every specific blood type. Subsequently, if you follow the same diet plan your next door neighbor is following; you may not be able to solve your weight issue the way s/he did; that diet may not be compatible with your body, and you will probably need to eat a different variety of foods I order to achieve your own weight loss goals.

This book will provide you with all the information you need in order to create a diet that matches your blood type. It will also clarify how you can take full advantage of the blood group specific foods in your quest for a better diet. By the time you finish reading this book, you will be able to successfully formulate a diet plan that revolves around your blood type, and that gives YOU maximum nutritional value.

Thanks again for downloading this book, I hope you enjoy it!

Chapter 1 - Good and bad foods based on blood type

Blood type diet revolves around the classification of foods to create diet that are blood type dependent. Dr. D'Adamo, the creator of this diet method, bases his theory about the evolution of blood groups on the work of the immunity chemist and blood type anthropologist William C. Boyd. After a worldwide survey, Boyd came up with a notion that our blood group variations have emerged with time as a part of evolution. In his 1950 book "Genetics and the races of man: An introduction to modern physical anthropology", he categorized the human population into 6 geographic distinctions. Later, in 1957, he increased the variations to up to 13 geographic distinctions. D'Adamo studied the association between the people of each group noted by Boyd and their blood groups, and finally came up with 4 different types of dietary plans for different ABO blood groups. Here is a highlight of these blood group specific plans:

- **'O' blood group** – referred to as **'the hunter'** by D'Adamo, and according to him thought to be the oldest blood type, originating some 30 thousand years back, has a dietary recommendation of protein rich diet. Foods that can be consumed by a type 'O' individual include lean meat, fish, poultry and vegetables. The individual should avoid grains, dairy and beans in their diet. Type 'O' people may experience stomach issues for which D'Adamo recommends supplements.

- **'A' blood group** – referred to as **'the cultivator'** or 'the agrarian', and originating some 20 millennia ago, when man first started to practice agriculture, has a recommended diet that is devoid of red meat and strictly vegetarian. People with this blood group should include plenty of vegetables, fruits, legumes, beans and whole grains in their diet. Basically, foods consumed by blood group 'A' individuals have to be fresh and organic since 'A' these individuals lack strong immune systems.

- **'B' blood group** – referred to as **'the nomad'**, and having arrived approximately 10 millennia ago. This blood group is linked to strong immunity and flexible digestion, which is why people with this blood group can benefit from dairy products. People with this blood type should eat green vegetables, specific meats, eggs and dairies that are low in fat content. They should stay clear of corn, buckwheat, wheat, lentils, peanuts, tomatoes and sesame seeds.

- **'AB' blood group** – referred to as **'the enigma'** is, according to D'Adamo, a very recent evolution that is only one millennium old. As the 'AB' name implies, this blood group has dietary recommendations that fall somewhere between those of blood group A and blood group B. Individuals with 'AB' blood type should consume a diet that is comprised of tofu, dairy, green vegetables and seafood. These individuals have lesser stomach acid, according to D'Adamo, which is why they should avoid alcohol and caffeine as well as cured/smoked meats.

Here is a chart that will provide you with a quick and easy reference when you are unsure whether a particular food is good for you:

Classification of diet according to blood type				
	Dietary Profile	Recommen ded completely	Recommen ded limitedly	Foods to stay clear of if you want to lose weight	Foods that you should eat to lose weight

'O' Type	Protein rich: Carnivorous	vegetables fruit Meat fish	grains legumes beans	wheat corn kidney beans navy beans lentils cabbage Brussels sprouts cauliflower mustard greens	kelp seafood salt liver red meat kale spinach broccoli
'A' Type	Vegan	vegetables grains beans tofu seafood legumes fruit		meat dairy lima beans wheat kidney beans	vegetable oil vegetables pineapple soy foods
'B' Type	Omnivorous	meat (except chicken) dairy beans legumes grains vegetables fruit		corn lentil seeds buckwheat peanuts sesame wheat	greens eggs licorice tea venison liver
'AB' Type	Moderately omnivorous	meat seafood beans legumes dairy tofu grains vegetables fruits		red meat kidney beans corn buckwheat lima beans seeds	tofu seafood kelp pineapple dairy greens

Chapter 2 - Why and how are foods given blood type classifications?

While working on the blood type analysis, Dr. Peter D'Adamo and his father Dr. James D'Adamo observed that many patients from European Spas who were on strict vegetarian diets or low fat diets did not lose weight. Following this lead, they followed more relevant studies, and finally came up with the idea that a person's blood type may be a factor that prevents certain diet plans from being successful. With investigation, their idea proved correct. For example, they found that people with blood type A did poorly on high protein diets, but did great when they were on vegetable proteins like Tofu and Soy. Curiously, the same diet plan did not work for people with blood type O; they did better with high protein diets and intense physical activities. These results encouraged the two doctors to come up with the idea of categorizing foods with different nutritional values according to their effects on people with different blood types. They wrote the details and findings of their work in the book *"Eat Right 4 Your Type"*.

Why are Certain Foods Incompatible with a Specific Blood Type?

The basic factor behind the blood grouping is the type of antigen present on the surface of the red blood cells; the antigens of the ABO blood group are sugars. A person's DNA determines the type of enzymes they have, and therefore, the type of sugar antigens that end up on their red blood cells. This, in turn, determines the blood group. Here is a look at different blood groups and their antigens:

Blood Group	Antigen Presented by RBC	Name of the Sugar Present
Blood Type A	A	Fucose and N-acetyl-galactosamine
Blood Type B	B	Fucose and D-galactosamine
Blood Type AB	A and B	Fucose, N-acetyl-galactosamine and D-galactosamine
Blood Type O	No Antigens	Only Fucose

The different sugars in different blood groups are responsible for the varying reactions to the same foods among individuals with different blood groups. According to an article published by the Vanderbilt University, the different sugar molecules present in different blood groups may interact with the different types of lectins present in food. However, these interactions will vary from one blood type to the other. For example, lectins that can cause harm to blood group A may not attack blood group O.

These chemical compounds known as lectins play a significant role in the reaction between foods and the blood. Lectins are abundantly and diversely present in dietary proteins, and they have the effect of agglutination on the blood. Agglutination, simply explained, is an effect in which the blood cells clump together. Basically, when you observe a diet that contains a type of lectins protein that is incompatible with your blood type antigen; there is a chance that these lectins can affect any organ in your body and cause blood cells to agglutinate together in the affected area. For example, milk lectins are more suitable for B blood group. Hence, if a person with Type A blood drinks milk, his/her system will immediately begin the agglutination process in order to reject it.

Although normal cooking destroys many lectins, others survive the cooking process. According to the researchers Gibbons and Dankers, from over 100 food plants containing active lectins, seven were found to be resistant to heat: apples, carrots, wheat bran, canned corn, pumpkin seeds, bananas, and wheat flour.

Another study conducted by Nachbar and Oppenheim noted that high levels of lectin activity are present in dry roasted peanuts, corn flakes, rice krispies, and Kelloggs Special K. They also found that the banana agglutinin was actually enhanced by heating. Another concern regarding lectins is their role in food allergies.

Consequences of the Hazardous Interactions between Blood type and Lectin

The lectins that escape the cooking process are the immune system's responsibility; it takes care of the majority of these lectins. Actually, around 95% of the lectins the body absorbs through diet are removed from the body. However, a minimum of 5% of the lectins consumed make their way into the blood stream and cause various reactions, some harmful, to occur in body organs. Common hazards of agglutination can include:

- Irritable bowel syndrome

- Cirrhosis of the liver

- Kidney problems

- Digestive problems

- A slowing of the rate of food metabolism

This is the reason why foods are categorized according to compatibility with blood type using a scientifically researched, logical and coherent plan that is based on cellular characteristics. When you follow this plan, you will be able to restore your intrinsic genetic pattern by consuming a strict diet that focuses on nutrients that are especially good for your blood type and that steers clear of the foods containing harmful lectins.

Chapter 3: Who is it for?

A blood type diet is not only useful for those looking to lose weight; it can be beneficial to almost anybody. Because the foods you eat react with your blood, following a diet specifically designed to match your blood type will help your body digest foods more efficiently. This simple change in diet can change your whole life, even if you are not looking to lose weight. Trying a blood type diet regimen will leave you feeling much better with an increased sense of wellbeing, heightened energy levels and increased immunity. With close investigation to the health benefits of a blood type diet, we can classify the individuals who would benefit from such a regimen into three groups of people.

1. People who are struggling with Their Body Weight

If your image in the mirror is seemingly increasing in size day after day, you are not alone. Obesity and over weight is a worldwide epidemic affecting 1.4 billion adults in different parts of the world, according to the World Health Organization

(WHO). These millions of individuals are striving to get their weight under control not only to address their self-image and self-confidence issues, but also to alleviate the hazardous health effects associated with excessive weight. People suffering from obesity are more prone to conditions such as cardiovascular disorders, diabetes, osteoarthritis and some cancers, according to the WHO.

Whether you had your health in mind, or were simply aiming to fit into that old pair of denim, you probably had your share of weight loss attempts. You may have already followed diet advice from doctors, dieticians or even from people who had a better luck trimming down their extra fat. If these efforts were mostly unsuccessful, and you're wondering about the reasons why, here is your answer. Traditional diet plans are mass produced as a one size fits all solution, which is a recipe for failure. Our bodies are different, and our approaches to change these bodies must differ accordingly in order to be met with success. Focusing on a person's blood type in the creation of a weight loss regimen does just that. Traditional diets overlook the dieter's blood type, although it is a very crucial factor in the digestion and metabolism of food. Ignoring this factor will result in a diet that is unsuitable for the individual needs of the dieter, and subsequently, unsatisfying results.

We have discussed how important it is to understand the chemistry taking place between your blood type and your weight in Chapter 5 - Blood type diet and weight loss. (**Go to Chapter 5**).

Feedback 65: This is an amazing program. I was eating lots of semolina pasta and I was morbidly obease! I was 270 June 1 1997, and on May 3rd, started this new programme. I have lost approximatly 25 pounds and I have not done any excersize yet!!! I am starting a new excersizing programme soon so I can really speed up my motabalism. My goal is to go from 270 pounds down to 190. I was starting out with a 44 inch waist and now I am down to a VERY loose 40. I hope to be a 36/34 inch waist! The last time I was a 34 waist was in Junior High School! I am truly happy!

If you are still confused about whether or not a blood type diet can help you in controlling your weight, you may like to read the following review. This review is written by a patient who had trouble with her obesity issue.

2. People who suffer from feelings of Stress and Weakness

Stress affects almost everybody in varying degrees. Experts recommend that you stop and rest whenever you feel stressed or weak, because stress is the body's way of alerting you to its increasing levels of fatigue (physical or mental), and its inability to cope with your current levels of activity without proper rest. In this sense, stress is a 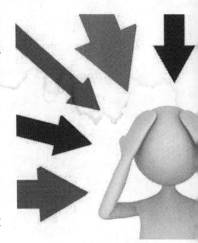 normal protective reaction from the body in order to shield itself from wearing out due to over exhaustion. However, if these feelings of stress and fatigue are recurrent, this means that you are not taking proper care of yourself, and that you need to look into the root of your stress problems or face the possible toll stress can take on your health in the forms of diabetes, gastrointestinal problems, depression, heart disease, obesity, asthma, neurodegenerative diseases like Alzheimer's disease, and even death.

To resolve unexplained and continuous stress and prevent it from recurring, you will need to have a balanced diet that is perfectly suitable for your individual needs, in addition to adopting an appropriate exercise routine. People with different blood types will need different stress management approaches as many studies have found a strong correlation between people's blood type and their behavior. Here are some effective examples suggested by Dr. Adamo for individuals with different blood groups that will help them reduce their stress levels:

Blood Type O: If your blood type is O, you are inheritably great at dealing with stress responses. However, prolonged stress may exhaust your brain which will affect your behavior negatively. If this happens, individuals with blood type O can show sudden rage with hyperactivity and even exert a manic episode. According to James D'Adamo, there is a powerful, synergistic relationship between the release of dopamine and feelings of reward; type O is more vulnerable to destructive behaviors when they are overwhelmed, tired, depressed or bored. The outcomes of these symptoms include gambling, sensation seeking, risk taking, substance abuse and impulsivity. If you are suffering from stress, a blood type diet can help you control your stress effectively, thus putting these symptoms under control and preventing them from recurring.

To get expert advice on how to control your stress by following a blood type diet and a suitable exercise routine, read **Chapter 4 - A model blood type diet plan**.

Blood Type A: Normally, individuals with blood type A have a high level of the stress hormone cortisol by nature. Put more simply, if your blood group is A, you are biologically more likely to face the hazards of prolonged stress. Some of these consequences are:

- Loss of energy due to muscle loss

- Sleep Disturbances

- Insulin Resistance

- Weight gain

- Obsessive-compulsive disorder (OCD)

- Hypothyroidism.

To get expert advice on how to control your stress by following a Bblood type diet and a suitable exercise routine, read **Chapter 4 - A model blood type diet plan**.

Blood Type B: Individuals with blood type B usually possess a perfectly balanced set of qualities. According to Dr. James D'Adamo, the dietary requirements of these individuals reflect this attribute. A proper and balanced combination of vegetables and animal protein is what gives these individuals the best results. However, as with type A, blood type B individuals also have higher levels of cortisol. Therefore, as a type B, you can get very upset when stressed. In addition, it may be hard for you to come out or recover from the effects of stress. This makes you prone to following stress related problems:

- Insulin Resistance

- Insomnia

- Daytime brain fog

- Gastrointestinal disturbances

- Reduced Immune response towards diseases

- Depression

- Hypothyroidism

In addition to the Cortisol problem, individuals with blood type B have an additional complication: rapid clearing of the

Nitric Oxide (NO). The Nitric Oxide molecule is a very important substance for the body as it affects many biological processes, including the nervous system and the immune system. Scientists have found that NO can enable the body to quickly recover from stress, possibly by regulating some neurotransmitters. They have also discovered that people with type B antigen appeared to clear NO more rapidly than people with other blood types. The reason for this is unknown, although one of the possible answers is the gene that influences the ability to modulate Arginine conversion into NO (nitric oxide) located right next to the gene that codes for blood type. The above problem may be the reason why it is so hard for you to feel alright after a long stretch of stressful activities.

You need not worry about these problems if you follow the blood type diet chart created by Dr. James D'Adamo. To get expert advice on how to control your stress by following a blood type diet and a suitable exercise routine, read <u>Chapter 4 - A model blood type diet plan</u>.

Blood Type AB: According to Dr. James D'Adamo, as a type AB individual, you may produce a high level of catecholamines like adrenaline. You also have the additional complexity of rapid clearing of nitrous oxide, just like type B individuals. You, therefore, have a very high chance to suffer from stress disorders. Individuals with blood type AB are naturally very considerate about others' feelings, and this leads them to hide their emotions on many occasions, especially when they feel angry or hostile. The damages resulting from repressing these feelings can cause more health problems than expressing anger would inflict. What diet can do to help with this problem is create a general sense of wellbeing that allows the individual to calm down and be at peace. By doing this, the body benefits from the reduced stress levels, and the individual is more likely to connect with his/her feelings and address this communication problem.

To get expert advice on how to control your stress by following a blood type diet and a suitable exercise routine, read Chapter 4 - A model blood type diet plan.

Feedback 8: The single greatest change in me since adopting the Type O eating plan has been a marked decrease in anxiety/panic. I attributed it to the reduction of the constant exhaustion/fatigue that was present when I was eating mainly Type A. I constantly avoided dairy products, along with the lectin in wheat- which is a major clogger/poison. I find I am able to eat much more food when I avoid wheat and dairy and still not gain weight. The seltzer water has also been a revelation, thanks again for your research.

If you are still confused about whether a blood type diet can help you to control your stress, you may like to read the following review. This review is written by a patient who had trouble with her anxiety and stress problems.

3. People Who Suffer from Blood Group Associated Diseases

You may have wondered why you suffer from certain health conditions in spite of taking every possible measure to live healthy. Have you ever considered your blood group to be a factor? It may be an unusual thing to believe, but the associations between blood group and certain health conditions have been established scientifically. For example, scientists have found that individuals with type A blood have a higher risk of Gastric Cancer, Hypercholesterolimia and Ischemic heart disease (Havlik, 1969). Those with blood type O were found to be more susceptible to Peptic ulcers and Hyperthyroidism (Villalobos 1990). As for individuals with blood type B, they were found to be more likely to have Anemia. Lastly, those with blood type AB are susceptible to heart diseases and bronchial infections (Muschel, 1966).

Based on research and documentation, Vanderbilt University has published the following list of diseases that may be linked to your blood type:

Type O	Type A	Type B	Type AB
Blood clotting disorders	Heart disease	Type I diabetes	Heart disease
Inflammatory diseases	Cancer	Chronic Fatigue Syndrome	Cancer
Low thyroid production	Anemia	Autoimmune disorders	Anemia
Ulcers	Liver and gallbladder disorders	Lou Gehrigs Disease	Bronchial infections
Allergies	Type I diabetes	Multiple Sclerosis	Parasitic infections

To learn more about the diseases that are associated with your blood group,

If you are still confused about whether a blood type diet can help you to control your blood type associated diseases, you may like to read the following review. This review is written by a patient who had trouble with her sinus problems for many years.

Chapter 4 - A model blood type diet plan

The Blood Type Diet has been popularized by the New York Times best seller 'Eat Right 4 Your Type' (ER4YT) written by Dr. James D'Adamo. This book has been translated into more than sixty languages over the course of ten years. If you are a blood type diet beginner in search of enough information to get started, you can follow the following models; they have been derived from that popular book and from references from other experts.

Model Blood Type Diet Plan for Blood Type O

As a type O individual, you are vulnerable to hyper-reactive immune responses, and are prone to digestive sensitivities. You will want to follow the following pieces of advice:

Eat According to Your Nutritional Needs:

- **Proteins:** Dr. Michael Lamand and Dr. James D'Adamo suggest that Type-O dieters should eat beef, lamb, turkey, chicken and fish. Bass, cod, halibut, sole and rainbow trout are good examples of fish that are suitable for individuals with blood type O, but fish like cod, herring and mackerel are also recommended. Type O individuals should avoid bacon, ham, goose, pork, catfish and smoked salmon.

- **Fats:** Type O individuals respond well to oils, according to Dr. James D'Adamo. You can, therefore, consume Olive oil, flaxseed oil, Canola oil and Sesame oil. However, Corn, Peanut and Cottonseed oils should be avoided.

- **Beans:** Beans, though high in fiber and protein, are not recommended for blood type O individuals. According to Dr. Lam, beans make muscle tissue less acidic and may even block the metabolism of other nutrients. If beans are included in the diet, Type O individuals should choose pinto beans or black-eyed peas.

- **Vegetables:** Garlic, kale, leeks, onions, red peppers, pumpkin and sweet potatoes are good vegetables for type O individuals. However, cruciferous vegetables like cabbage, Brussels sprouts, cauliflower and mustard greens should be avoided because they inhibit thyroid functions. Eggplants and potatoes are also not recommended because it is believed that they contribute to arthritis. Corn should be avoided as well as it adversely affects insulin regulation in the body.

- **Fruits:** Plums, prunes, figs and limited amounts of grapefruit are the only fruits type O individuals should eat. Highly acidic fruits like oranges and strawberries may irritate the stomach lining. Additionally, melons and cantaloupes tend to have high mold counts, which may lead to allergy problems.

- **Drinks:** Type O individuals should drink plenty of water, seltzer water, club soda and tea. Beer and wine are fine in moderation. However, coffee, distilled liquors and black teas should be avoided. Caffeine can be particularly harmful because of its tendency to raise adrenaline and noradrenaline; both of which are already high in the bodies of individuals with blood type O.

- **Dairy:** Dairy products that can trigger digestive malfunctions should be avoided.

Make Time for Exercise:

Regular exercise is an effective stress relief tool, especially aerobic activities such as biking, running or hiking. Choose one of these activities and perform it for 30 to 45 minutes, at least four times per week. If you are easily bored, choose two or three different exercises and vary your routine. This, in addition to your new blood type diet, is guaranteed to result change in both your body and wellbeing.

Model Blood Type Diet Plan for Blood Type A

To help balance the high cortisol levels of blood type A individuals, Dr. James D'Adamo recommends a combination of vegetable prioritized diet and exercise. "I can't emphasize enough how this critical dietary adjustment can be to the sensitive immune system of Type A. With this diet you can supercharge your immune system and potentially short circuit the development of life threatening diseases," says Dr. James

D'Adamo. Here is a condensed version of his advice to individuals with blood type A:

Eat According to Your Nutritional Needs:

- **Proteins:** Fish and poultry should be limited in the diet of individuals with blood type A, because their bodies produce fewer meat-digesting enzymes causing them to have a hard time digesting meats, especially red meats. To get their daily requirement of proteins, they should rely on plant protein from nuts and nut butters, seeds, beans and soy. A more savory protein that is recommended for blood type A individuals is specific seafood such as mahi-mahi, cod, mackerel, sea bass, carp, pike, red snapper, salmon, sturgeon, tuna, sardine, perch, tilapia and shark. However, they should avoid squid, barracuda, clam, crab, lobster, trout, shrimp and octopus.

- **Vegetables:** Broccoli, artichokes, carrots, greens, garlic and almost all vegetables are good for blood type A individuals. Unrecommended vegetables, however, include cabbage, eggplant and tomatoes; those should be consumed in limited amounts.

- **Fruits:** Blood type A individuals should eat berries, figs, plums, apples, avocados, pears and peaches.

- **Drinks:** Sugar, caffeine and alcohol are allowed, but only in limited amounts.

- **Other:** It is recommended that individuals with blood type A eat smaller but more frequent meals in order to help stabilize blood sugar levels.

- **Recommended nutritional supplements for blood type A:**

    Vitamin B12- Since individuals with blood type A have a thinner gastric layer than others due to low stomach acids, they may have difficulty in absorbing Vitamin B12. They should take supplement containing B12 to avoid its deficiency.

    Vitamin C – They should also eat plenty of fruits that contain vitamin C, or alternately get their Vitamin C requirements through a supplement. Vitamin C is particularly useful at reversing the ill-effects of nitrites found in smoked/cure meats to which blood type A individuals are particularly susceptible.

    Calcium – Calcium requires high stomach acid levels to be digested properly, so blood type A individuals are at a disadvantage here. Aside from dairy, the best foods for you to derive calcium from are eggs, goat milk, broccoli and spinach. You can take calcium tablets if you are unable to obtain the proper amount of calcium through nutrition.

Iron – Unfortunately, those with blood type A cannot use red meats as a source of iron, since they don't digest it very well. The best iron-rich foods for them are beans, figs, and blackstrap molasses. Iron supplements are a good option as they help blood type A individuals in maintaining their iron levels.

Make Time for Exercise:

For blood type A, Dr. James D'Adamo recommends Hatha Yoga, Tai Chi, Meditation and Deep Breathing Exercises. Meditation has been studied for its effects on stress hormones, and it was found that after meditation, serum Cortisol levels were significantly reduced. Meditation can also help in the control of Nitrous oxide which relieves stress symptoms.

Model Blood Type Diet Plan for Blood Type B

People with Type B blood are able to digest a wide range of foods, but they may need to avoid some of these foods nevertheless, to avoid weight gain. Here are some Do's and Don'ts from Dr. James D'Adamo to blood type B individuals:

Eat According to Your Nutritional Needs:

- **Proteins:** Get your protein from goat, lamb, mutton, rabbit and venison. Avoid eating too much chicken as it contains a blood type B agglutinating lectin in its muscle tissue. Although chicken is a lean meat, the issue is the power of an agglutinating lectin attacking your bloodstream and the potential for it to lead to strokes and immune disorders.

- **Vegetables**: Eat plenty of leafy greens and vegetables.

- **Fruits:** Bananas, grapes, plums and pineapple can be really good for you.

- **Dairy:** Consume low fat dairy.

- **Other:** Corn, wheat, buckwheat, lentils, tomatoes, peanuts and sesame seeds should be eaten only in limited amounts as they can contribute to weight gain, fatigue, fluid retention, and hypoglycemia.

Make Time for Exercise:

Dr. James D'Adamo recommends that people with blood type B choose physical exercises that challenge the mind as well as the body. They need to balance meditative activities with more intense physical exercise such as tennis, martial arts, cycling, hiking and golf. "You tend to do best with activities that are not too aerobically intense, have an element of mental challenge and involve other people," says Dr. James D'Adamo. This means that you can work on your fitness and have fun with friends at the same time!

Model Blood Type Diet Plan for Blood Type AB

If your blood type is AB, your body will need a vegetable-rich diet with a variety of carbohydrates. Since you have a slightly alkaline stomach, you might have a hard time digesting acidic foods like oranges. Below are some tips for those with blood type AB that will help them manage their diets and obtain a healthier lifestyle.

Eat According to Your Nutritional Needs:

- **Proteins:** Those with blood type AB can eat turkey, goat, lamb, liver, mutton, ostrich, pheasant and rabbit. Protein containing foods they should avoid are beef, bacon, ham, chicken, duck, goose, partridge, quail, veal and venison. As for seafood, mahimahi, cod, grouper, mackerel, bluefish, carp, caviar, pike, red snapper, salmon, sturgeon, tuna, scallop, sardine, mussel, all kinds of perch, herring, tilapia, catfish, shark and squid are all suitable for blood type B individuals. However, bass, barracuda, clam, crab, lobster, oyster, trout, shrimp and conch should be avoided.

- **Dairy and eggs**: Individuals with blood type AB can safely eat cottage, farmer and cream cheeses, but they should avoid American and blue cheeses. They can also eat feta, Mozzarella, ghee, casein, milk, eggs (all but duck), ricotta and all kinds of yogurt. It is preferable that they stay away from butter, ice cream and parmesan cheese.

- **Oils and fats:** Olives and walnuts are good for those with blood type AB. These individuals can also eat almond, black currant seed, borage seed, canola oil, peanut, soy, wheat germ and cod liver. However, they should try to avoid eating coconut, safflower, sesame and sunflower.

- **Nuts and seeds:** Chestnuts, peanuts peanut butter and walnuts are the safest options for AB blood type individuals. They can also eat almond butter and cashew. However, Hazelnuts, poppy seeds, pumpkin seeds, sesame butter and seeds, sunflower butter and seeds are not suitable for this blood type.

- **Beans and Legumes:** Lentil, navy bean, pinto bean, soybean, soy miso, cannellini bean, soy tofu, green or snap or string beans are great options for those with blood type AB. They can also eat peas, soy cheese, soy milk, tamarind beans and white beans. The beans and legumes they should try to avoid are black eyed peas, lima beans, fava beans and mung beans or sprouts.

- **Vegetables:** The recommended vegetables for AB blood type are alfalfa, sprouts, beet greens and beet, broccoli, cauliflower and celery. They can also eat Arugua, asparagus, bamboo shoot, cabbage, caraway, okra, olive (green, Greek, Spanish), onion, potato, pumpkin, cucumber, eggplant, garlic, kale, mustard greens, parsley, chicory, cilantro, fennel, ginger, seaweeds, spinach, squash, tomato and lettuce. Vegetables that are not very suitable for their digestion are Aloe, caper, black olives, pepper, pickles, radish and rhubarb.

- **Fruits:** Cherry, cranberry, fig, gooseberry, grape. Apple, apricot, Asian pear, black and blueberry, papaya, peach, pear, kiwi, lemon, pineapple, plum, watermelon, cantaloupe and dates are all examples of the fruits recommended for blood type AB. The fruits that should be avoided are avocado, banana, coconut, guava, mango, orange, persimmon, pomegranate, quince and starfruit.

Make Time for Exercise:

Dr. James D'Adamo recommends a combination of both calming activities and more intense physical exercise; this helps to maintain an optimal balance. For example, you can dedicate three days to aerobic exercise such as running or biking, and two days for calming exercise such as yoga or tai chi.

Chapter 5 - Blood type diet and weight loss

Has the long, grueling, seemingly endless struggle to lose weight been tormenting you for years and years? If so, you may have found the way out of this frustrating tunnel. Follow the blood type diet instructions; eat the foods that individually suit your blood type, and exercise regularly according to the instructions provided in the previous chapter. If you do this, you will probably never have to worry about your weight again. There are only two steps in this weight loss process:

Step 1: Know about foods that are beneficial for you. Many weight loss diet plans can ruin your health, weaken your muscle, and even those who don't are not likely to give you the results you need. Closely examine the blood type diet models in the previous chapter and take notes of the recommended and un-recommended foods for your blood type.

Step 2: Start following the plan slowly, gradually building up the momentum needed to follow your individual plan accurately. Remember that you cannot change damage that has taken years to happen overnight, so you need to be patient. The first results you will notice will be with your digestion and your sense of wellbeing and energy levels. Changes to your body will soon follow if you keep adhering to your plan. Just like with dieting, start exercise slowly, especially if you haven't worked out in a while; there is no need to strain your body and subject it to injury in the first week. Let your body get accustomed to your new habits slowly.

Blood Type Diet Individualization for Weight Control

Blood Type O

If your blood type is O, you should feel honored; you have the most ancient blood group of human history. From your ancestors, you have got the characteristics of a great hunter; hunting animals is what kept the humans alive back then. You are highly focused, energetic and very realistic. You can get things done. However, to keep going strong at your high level of energy, you need to eat plenty of protein and do vigorous exercises; just like an ancient hunter! A diet that does not suit you and/or a life style that lacks physical activity can hamper your metabolic effects and **lower your thyroid hormone**. Iodine deficiency as a result of a poor diet can also lead to lowered levels of thyroid hormones, which may lead you to feel weak and gain weight.

If you are a blood type O individual eating a seemingly healthy vegetable rich diet, and still suffering from weight gain, the above explanation could be the root of your problem, and you will to increase the amount of protein in your diet. According to Dr. James D'Adamo, instead of treating the iodine deficiency with an Iodine supplement, you should correct your hormone regulation. You should adopt a diet rich in saltwater fish, which will help your body to regulate the thyroid gland. The sea weed Bladder Wrack can also be an excellent nutrient for type O's as it is very effective as an aid to weight control for Type O's. "The fucose in bladder wrack seems to help normalize the sluggish metabolic rate and produce weight loss in Type O's," says Dr. James D'Adamo.

Short Note for Blood Type O

Foods that will cause weight gain and should be avoided: Wheat gluten, corn, kidney beans, navy beans, lentils, cabbage, Brussels sprouts, cauliflower and mustard greens.

Foods that will help you to lose weight: Kelp, Seafood, Iodized salt, kale, liver, spinach and broccoli.

Blood Type A

If you your blood type is A, you have a very interesting history; instead of sticking with hunting animals to provide food, your ancestors invented agriculture turning humans from simple wanderers into more civilized beings who know how to cope with changing conditions.

The cultivation of grains and livestock is a very important part of our history. It is because of it that people were able to build stable communities for the first time. What does this say about you as a blood type A individual? Like your ancestors, you also have the quality of a genius; you can use any available resource to your 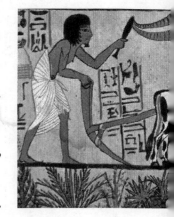 benefit. You also have a great connection between your mind and your body. In a study conducted by Dr. James D'Adamo in 1999, he found that people with blood type A have great qualities; they were shown to be details oriented, analytical, creative, inventive, good listeners, and very sensitive to the needs of others.

According to the findings of Dr. James D'Adamo, people with blood type A have the need to fully utilize nutrients from carbohydrate sources. These biological adaptations can still be observed today in type A's digestive structure. People with this blood group will have low levels of hydrochloric acid in the stomach and high intestinal disaccharide digestive enzyme. These enzymes are best for the digestion of carbohydrates. On the other hand, the same individuals will have low levels of intestinal alkaline phosphatase, which makes it difficult for type A individuals to digest and metabolize animal protein and fat. This is why blood type A individuals are recommended to eat large amounts of vegetables in order to live a healthy life and control their weight.

Short Note for Blood Type A

Foods that will cause weight gain and should be avoided: Dairy, kidney beans, wheat, and lima beans.

Foods that will help you to lose weight: Vegetable oils, soy foods, vegetables and pineapple.

Blood Type B

If your blood type is B, you have the most balanced qualities of nature. Your blood type has evolved after both "O" group and "A" group. Your blood type makes humans more capable of utilizing natural resources. According to the studies conducted by Dr. James D'Adamo and other researchers, you

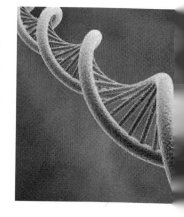

are creative, original, and flexible. Researchers also noted that you are a great student of nature; you learn through observation and you proceed to make the right decision afterwards.

Blood Type B developed in the area of the Himalayan highlands, now part of present day Pakistan and India, mainly because people wanted to settle down in a friendly climate. Anthropologists are suspecting that blood type B may have initially been a mutation in response to climactic changes. This blood group first appeared in India or the Ural region of Asia among a mix of Caucasian and Mongolian tribes. At this time, you could see this new blood group mostly in Europeans and Asians. After this, the Mongolians moved northward and started farming and domesticating animals. They later adopted a diet consisting of meat, milk and other dairy products along with vegetables.

Like your ancestors, you have a highly sophisticated gene developed to utilize the best nutrition possible. However, according to Dr. James D'Adamo, these genes which are closer to the ABO blood type gene may affect your stomach acid levels. To take care of your health, you will need to consume both vegetables and protein at a balanced rate. If you don't eat the right kinds of food, you may have an increased cortisol level, which increases your stress level and, indirectly, your body weight. According to Dr. James D'Adamo, people with blood type B are very successful in controlling their body weight; all they need is perfect balance and harmony in their lifestyle and diet.

Short Note for Blood Type B

Foods that will cause weight gain and should be avoided: Corn, peanuts, wheat, sesame seeds, and lentils.

Foods that will help you to lose weight: Meat, liver, eggs, licorice tea and green Vegetables.

Blood Type AB

If your blood type is AB, you are one of the very unique; only 5 % of the world population shares your blood type. Blood type AB started appearing in humans in the last ten or twelve centuries. AB blood type is composed of the properties of blood groups A and B. It, therefore, possesses both of these types' merits and demerits. As an individual with blood 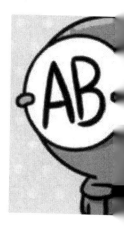 type AB, you are emotional, passionate, friendly, trusting and very sociable. You are not very prone to gaining excess weight, because your body is developed to tune up with your eating pattern. Nevertheless, there are certain things you will want to keep in mind when it comes to your diet and lifestyle.

"Type AB has Type A's low stomach acid, however, they also have Type B's adaptation to meats. Therefore, you lack enough stomach acid to metabolize them efficiently and the meat you eat tends to get stored as fat. Your Type B propensities cause the same insulin reaction as Type B when you eat lima beans, corn, buckwheat, or sesame seeds," says famous naturopath Dr. James D'Adamo. He suggests that type AB avoid combining certain foods. For example, type AB individuals will digest and metabolize foods more efficiently if they avoid eating starches and proteins in the same meal.

Short Note for Blood Type AB

Foods that will cause weight gain and should be avoided: Red meat, kidney beans, lima beans, corn, wheat and seeds.

Foods that will help you to lose weight: Tofu, dairy, kelp, pineapple and green Vegetables.

Chapter 6 - Blood type diet recipes

Once you have made a list of the foods that are good for your blood type, making meals that suit these dietary requirements is very easy. You can turn your kitchen into a cooking laboratory, and have fun with new food combination every day!

Although cooking experimentation is very fun, there is no doubt that you are going to need a quick easy recipe to carry you through those busy days.

Below are easy to cook recipes that are suitable for all blood types (A, B, O, and AB), and are also very delicious! Bon Appetite!

Appetizer

Delicious Egg recipe with Onion, Black Pepper and Spinach

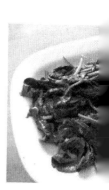

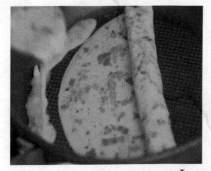 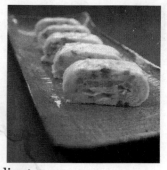

2 eggs
1 handful of Spinach
1 teaspoon of finely chopped onion
1 teaspoon of finely chopped Parsley
1 teaspoon of finely chopped carrot
Black pepper to taste
Salt to taste

Preparation

1. In a bowl, mix two eggs with onions, black pepper, salt, carrot and parsley
2. Pour some olive or soy oil into the pan, sauté the egg mixture in the pan, roll it up with a spoon, and then place the roll on the pan when done.
3. Put the Spinach in the pan and steam it for a while. When done, add a little olive oil on top of it.
4. Serve the egg roll along with the steamed Spinach.

Main Meal

Salsa & Salmon (Blood Type Friendly Version)

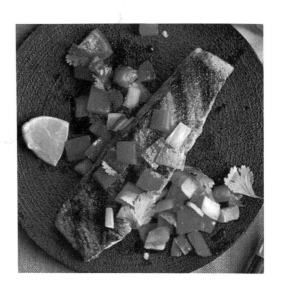

Ingredients

Salmon
2 teaspoons of black pepper or chili powder
1 teaspoon ground cumin
1/2 teaspoon salt
1/2 teaspoon ground coriander
4 skinless salmon fillets (About 6 ounces in total)
Cooking spray

Salsa

1/4 cup chopped tomato or broccoli or carrot
¼ cup chopped green capsicum
2 tablespoons pre-chopped red onion
1 tablespoon chopped fresh cilantro
1 1/2 teaspoons fresh lime juice
1/8 teaspoon salt

Preparation

1. To prepare the salmon, heat a grill pan over medium-high heat. Combine the first 5 ingredients and rub them evenly over fillets.
2. Coat the pan with cooking spray.
3. Add fillets to pan; cook 4 minutes on each side or until desired degree of doneness.
4. While the fish cooks, prepare the salsa. If you are going to use carrot or broccoli, then boil the vegetable for a small amount of time.
5. Serve salsa with fillets.

Broiled Tuna

Ingredients:

1 can solid white tuna, canned in water
1 tablespoon mayonnaise
1 teaspoon mustard
2 scallions, minced
3 rice cakes
3 tablespoons shredded mozzarella
A sprinkle of Season-All Salt

Preparation:

1. Mash the tuna to break up large chunks.
2. Mix together well with the mayonnaise and mustard.
3. Stir in scallions.

4. Divide the mixture among rice cakes and spread evenly to cover entire rice cake.
5. Top with shredded mozzarella
6. Broil until cheese melts and turns golden.
7. Sprinkle lightly with salt.
8. Serves 3 for lunch or snack.

Meat Loaf for all Blood Types

Ingredients:

Olive oil spray
1/2 cup onion, thinly sliced
1/2 cup carrots, thinly sliced
1/2 cup mushrooms, thinly sliced [omit for type A-non & O]
2 roasted nori (dried seaweed leaves), torn into small pieces
3/4 pound ground white meat turkey
1 egg white
sea salt and freshly ground black pepper (Type O)
Tomato sauce
1/2 cup Contadina tomato paste
1/2 cup water
1/4 cup diced onions
2 cloves garlic crushed

Preparation

1. Preheat oven to 400 degrees Fahrenheit.
2. Line a baking sheet with parchment paper, and spray with olive oil spray.
3. Heat a nonstick skillet, and coat with olive oil spray.
4. Add onions, carrots and mushrooms and sauté for five minutes.
5. Mix vegetables with roasted nori, ground turkey and egg white.
6. Add sea salt & pepper to taste.

7. Divide ground turkey into two portions, place both portions on a baking tray, and shape into two loaves about 6' x 3.'
8. Bake for 15 minutes. Makes two servings.

The following topping can be prepared while the turkey meat loaf cooks.

Vermont (type A)

1. Mix 3 tablespoons of maple syrup with 3 teaspoons of Dijon mustard.
2. Spoon the sauce over the top when the meat loaf is finished baking.

Salad

Greek Salad

Ingredients:

1 head romaine/leaf lettuce or spinach

1 cucumber sliced [optional]

1/2 cup feta cheese

Lemon Dressing

1/4 cup olive oil

2 tablespoons lemon juice

1 tablespoons Dijon mustard

1/2 teaspoon sugar [or agave]

Sea salt and pepper to taste

Preparation

1. Combine torn lettuce or spinach with sliced cucumber, and top with feta cheese.

2. Meanwhile combine dressing ingredients and shake well.

3. Pour the dressing over the salad and toss.

Dessert

Banana & Pear with Almond Milk

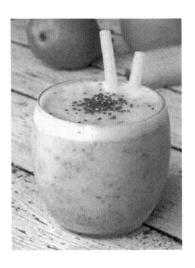

Ingredients

1 frozen banana, peeled
1 cup almond milk (refrigerated)
½ pear
Chia seeds (not mandatory)

Preparation

1. Put all the ingredients in a blender

2. Blend all ingredients well
3. Pour into a cup and enjoy!

Delicious Egg recipe with Onion, Black Pepper and Spinach

Ingredients

2 eggs
1 handful of Spinach
Finely chopped onions 1 tsp
Finely chopped Parsley 1 spoon full
Finely chopped carrot 1 tsp
Black pepper as per wish
Salt as per wish

Instructions

· In a bowl, mix two eggs with onions, black pepper, salt, carrot and parsley

· Pour some olive or Soy oil on the pan, sauté the egg mixture in the pan, roll it up with spoon and then place the roll on the pan when done.

· Pour Spinach on the pan, steam it for a while, when done add a little olive oil on it.

· Serve the egg roll along with the steamed Spinach on the plate and enjoy

Pineapple Cake

Ingredients

1/4 cup maple sugar [or BTD compliant sweetener]
3/4 cup oat flour [or BTD compliant flour]
3/4 cup rice flour
1 teaspoon baking powder
1 teaspoon baking soda
1/8 teaspoon sea salt
1/3 cup oil
3/4 cup maple syrup
2/3 cup tofu, pureed
1/4 cup pineapple juice
1 tablespoon vanilla
2 tablespoon lemon juice
1 can pineapple rings (10 ounce can)

Preparation

1. Preheat oven to 350 degrees F.

2. Coat baking pan with cooking spray.

3. Sprinkle with maple sugar.

4. Place pineapple rings on top of maple sugar, so the rings touch each other and line the pan.

5. In a large bowl sift together flour, baking powder, baking soda and salt.

6. In another bowl, whisk together oil, maple syrup, tofu, pineapple juice, vanilla and lemon juice.

7. Pour wet ingredients into dry ingredients and mix lightly with wire whisk.

8. Don't over mix; batter will be heavy.

9. Pour batter into pan and bake for 25 to 35 minutes.

10. When done, invert pan onto plate.

Individualized Blood Type Diet Recipes

For Type O and B

Mushroom and Beef Roast

Ingredients

1/2 teaspoon salt
1/4 teaspoon pepper, freshly ground
2 pounds flank steak
1 teaspoon Dijon mustard
2 tablespoons olive oil
1 cup onion, chopped
4 ounces Portobello mushrooms, chopped
1/4 cup parsley, chopped
2 tablespoons chives, chopped
1 tablespoon tomato paste (This should be overlooked for blood type
B individuals)
1/4 cup Ezekiel or spelt bread crumbled fine
1/4 teaspoon salt
1/4 teaspoon pepper
1 teaspoon paprika
3 strips turkey bacon (This should be overlooked for blood type B
individuals)
2 each onion, chopped
A 10 ounce can of beef broth
1 teaspoon Dijon mustard
2 tablespoons acceptable catsup

Preparation

1. Lightly salt and pepper flank steak on both sides. Coat one side with mustard.

2. To prepare stuffing, heat vegetable oil in a fry pan, add 1 onion, chopped, and cook for 3 minutes, until lightly browned.

3. Chop canned mushroom pieces.

4. Add to onion, and cook for 5 minutes.

5. Stir in parsley, chives, tomato paste, and bread crumbs. Season with salt, pepper and paprika.

6. Spread stuffing on mustard side of flank steak, and roll it up jelly-roll fashion. Tie with string or a toothpick.

7. Dice bacon. To prepare gravy, cook bacon in Dutch oven until partially done (you will probably need to add a little olive oil because there's almost no fat in turkey bacon).

8. Add the meat roll and brown on all sides for approximately 10 minutes.

9. Add the other 2 chopped onions and sauté for 5 minutes.

10. Pour in beef broth, cover, and simmer for 1 hour.

11. Remove meat when tender.

12. Season pan juices w/mustard.

13. Add salt and pepper to taste, and stir in catsup (or tomato paste).

14. When meat is slightly cooled, slice into 8 pieces and place in 2 ziplocs.

15. Cool sauce, freeze in 2 Ziplocs with meat slices.

16. Thaw, reheat meat and gravy separately.

Yummy Chicken Mix

Ingredients

4 chicken breasts [or other BTD compliant protein]
1/2 cup olive oil mayonnaise [or other BTD compliant mayo]

1/4 cup non-dairy sour cream (optional)
2-3 cloves of garlic (minced)
1/2 a medium onion (minced)
2 tablespoons chopped fresh parsley
1/4 cup chopped walnuts
1 cup red grapes (cut in half)
1 pinch fresh dill (optional)
Chili powder (to taste)

Preparation

1. Boil Chicken Breasts till cooked through, but still firm. Cool.

2. Combine all ingredients mixing thoroughly, but try to keep the chicken in chunks.

3. Chill and serve over lettuce or allowable crackers.

Spicy Lamb curry

Ingredients

2 pounds stewed lamb
1 cup onion, finely chopped
1 tablespoon oil
1/8 teaspoon cayenne or more
1/2 teaspoon coriander, ground
3 tablespoons curry powder or to taste
1/2 cup chicken broth (substitute with turkey broth for blood group B)

Preparation

1. Defrost the Stewed Lamb if frozen.

2. Combine the onions, oil, cayenne, coriander and curry powder in a 2-quart saucepan over medium heat.
3. Cook while stirring continuously for 2 minutes.
4. Add the broth and cook for another 2 minutes.
5. Add the lamb and sauce. Reduce the heat to low, cover, and cook until bubbling hot (about 25 minutes).
6. Remove the pan from the heat, transfer the mixture to a serving dish, and serve immediately.
7. If your curry is very hot, serve a side dish of plain yogurt with your chicken curry (only allowed for blood type B)

For Type A and AB

Asian Flavored Tempeh

Ingredients

1 package of Tempeh sliced in half and cut into bite sized pieces
MARINADE
1/4 cup Tamari (wheat free soy sauce)
1 clove of Garlic (more if you want)
1 teaspoon of fresh ground Ginger (more for a spicy taste)
Juice of half a lemon (more if you want)
1 teaspoon of olive oil

Preparation

1. Boil a pot of water.
2. Slice tempeh in half, and then slice further into bite size pieces.
3. Once the water is boiling, drop the tempeh in and set the timer for 5 minutes.
4. While the tempeh is boiling get your marinade ready.

5. Drain the tempeh, add to the marinade and refrigerate in a container for a few hours or overnight. (It is better to use a glass container, rather than plastic).

6. Every time you open the fridge, shake the container to move the marinade around.

7. Cook briefly in a skillet to heat and brown a bit.

8. Serve over rice or other grain.

Chicken Lasagna

Ingredients

1/2 cup ghee
1/2 cup spelt flour
1/2 teaspoon sea salt
1/2 teaspoon basil
3 cups chicken broth
2.5 cups cooked chicken, cubed
1 pint ricotta cheese
1 egg, slightly beaten
8 ounces rice lasagna noodles, cooked
10 ounce package frozen (or fresh) chopped spinach, thawed, well-drained
4 ounces mozzarella cheese, thinly sliced
1/4 cup Parmesan cheese, grated

Preparation

1. Melt ghee in a medium sized saucepan.

2. Blend in flour, salt and basil.

3. Stir in chicken broth and cook, stirring constantly, until mixture thickens and comes to a boil.

4. Remove from heat.

5. Add chicken.

6. Combine ricotta cheese with egg, and mix well.

7. In a greased 13x9 inch baking dish, place 1/3 of chicken mixture.

8. Layer half the noodles, half the ricotta cheese mixture, half the spinach and all the mozzarella cheese.

9. Repeat, ending with the last 1/3 of chicken.

10. Top with Parmesan cheese.

11. Bake at 375 Fahrenheit for 45 minutes.

12. Serves 6.

Chicken Chili

Ingredients

1 tablespoon flour (can substitute with millet or brown rice)
2 tablespoons instant minced onion
1 tablespoon chili powder (if you don't like spicy food, substitute with 1-2 teaspoons of cumin powder)
1 teaspoon salt
1/4 teaspoon red pepper (optional)
1/2 teaspoon instant minced garlic (see note below for onion and garlic changes)
1/2 teaspoon ground cumin
1 pound lean ground meat (beef or turkey or chicken)
2 * 15.5 ounce cans great northern beans
2 cups water
Chili Seasoning, the whole amount above
2 stalks celery, chopped

Note: To replace the instant onion and garlic in the seasoning mix with fresh ingredients use:

1 chopped onion
1 minced clove of garlic
Brown these with the meat

1. Brown your ground meat of choice (beef or turkey or chicken) over medium heat, in a deep medium to big sized.
2. If using fresh onions and garlic, add them to the ground meat and brown.
3. Drain, if desired.
4. Add beans, water, seasoning mix, and celery.
5. Bring to a simmer, reduce heat to medium low, and allow to cook for about 30 minutes, or until desired thickness is reached, stirring occasionally.

Lime Fish with Sea Salt

Ingredients

4 to 6 large fillets of any Neutral/beneficial white fish
Juice of two limes or lemons
Fresh ginger cut into thin slices
6 to 8 cloves of garlic, crushed
Sea salt, to taste

Preparation

1. Preheat your oven to 350 degrees Fahrenheit.
2. Place the fish on large piece of tin foil.
3. Pour juice of lemon or lime over fish.
4. Place ginger and limes slices over fish and sprinkle with crushed garlic and sea salt.
5. Completely wrap the fish in the tin foil so none of the juice(s) can escape.

6. Place the fish wrapped in the aluminum on a flat cookie tray and place in the oven.
7. Bake for 20 to 30 minutes.
8. Check for doneness by slowly opening the foil and poking the fish with a fork. Be careful when you open the foil wrap and keep your hands away from the arising steam to avoid burns.

From the Kitchen of a Vegetarian

Vegetarianism have always been viewed as the healthy option. It is true that vegetables are some of the healthiest things a person can eat; packed full of vitamins and minerals and low on caloric content as they are. Your blood type may have a say on whether or not vegetarianism will be as healthy for your body as you may think.

If your blood type is A, and you are living a vegetarian lifestyle, you are definitely on the right track. Individuals with blood type O, however, are highly unlikely to accomplish their health and weight loss goals on a vegetarian diet. Not only will they fail to lose weight, they may also become weak, de-energized and sick. Below is a type O vegetarian customer review on dadamo.com.

"
  I have gradually worked my way into this diet (Blood Type Diet). Before I began, I was an overweight, fatigued vegetarian, and constantly coming down with various illnesses. After hearing and reading a bit about the diet, I began eating meats (particularly lean reds and fish), and modified my other eating habits according to the plan. Over the past year and one half (when I began modifying my diet), I have had no significant illnesses, I've lost weight, I have constant energy, and I have a better sense of well being. I have even felt a greater hormonal drive. My life has really taken a 360 degree turn since I began
  "
the diet.

As for people with blood types B and AB, following a vegetarian diet can be compatible with their goals, but they will be better off by adding some fish protein to their diets. The best practice for these individuals would be to eat plenty of vegetables and frequently add other types of foods that are recommended for their blood types. Here are some popular recipes for vegetarians you may like to try:

Green Beets and Onion Mix

Ingredients

Two bunches of beet greens including whole stems

Goat feta or sprinkle powder cheese, to taste
Granulate garlic, to taste
Onion, to taste

Preparation

1. Steam all the greens, stems included, in a little water over medium heat until tender but not overcooked.
2. Slice the stems & greens into bite size pieces.
3. Add goat feta or sprinkle powder cheese.
4. Add a granulated garlic and/or onion to taste.

Note: never add salt, it has enough of its own.

Banana Carrot Cake

Ingredients

1/4 pounds butter, chopped (can be substituted with ghee)
1 cup sugar (can be substituted with brown sugar, maple sugar, agave syrup)
1 egg, lightly beaten
1 medium carrot, coarsely grated
2 over ripe bananas, mashed
1.5 cups rice flour
1 teaspoon baking soda
1 teaspoon allspice (blood groups B and AB should substitute this with nutmeg)
3/4 cup walnuts or pecans, chopped

1/4 teaspoon baking powder

Preparation

1. Cream butter and sugar in the mixer.
2. Add the egg and beat until combined.
3. Add carrots and bananas.
4. Add sifted dry ingredients and nuts, stirring until combined.
5. Spread into prepared 8 inch pan or ring pan.
6. Place in a preheated oven on 350 degrees Fahrenheit, and bake for about 1 hour or until a skewer comes out clean.
7. Let the cake cool for at least 5 minutes before taking it out of the pan.

Vegan Noodles

Ingredients

Onions
Garlic
Sea salt
Chopped celery
Diced collard green
One big bunch of diced parsley
2 to 3 strips of turkey bacon
Olive oil
Ghee
Rice noodles
1 cup water
Coriander
A pinch of black pepper

Preparation

1. Sauté all the vegetables in the olive oil.
2. Add salt. Stir well and often for 5 – 10 minutes.
3. Add 1 cup of water and one package of Thai rice noodles (any rice noodle will do).
4. Throw in one big tablespoon of ghee (optional).
5. The Thai noodles cook up in about 6 minutes.
6. When noodles are ready, season with more salt, pepper and coriander seed.
7. Serve with sliced gala apples on the side.

Vegan lasagna

Ingredients

3 tablespoons olive oil
1 red pepper, chopped
2 teaspoons basil
1 teaspoon oregano
2 bay leaves
1 teaspoon salt
1/2 a can tomato paste
1 can chopped tomato
1 large fresh tomato, chopped
2 tablespoons red wine
6 rice lasagna noodles (Tinkyada brand recommended)
1 * 14 ounce block firm tofu
1 egg
2 teaspoons soy sauce
1 teaspoon apple cider vinegar
16 ounces soft mozzarella cheese (or 12 ounces regular mozzarella)
1/2 cup goat cheese

1. Sauté pepper in oil for 5 minutes with herbs and salt.
2. Add tomato sauce, tomato paste, fresh tomatoes and wine.
3. Simmer for 45 minutes.
4. Meanwhile, cook rice noodles according to package directions.
5. Squeeze tofu in a soft cloth until all water is squeezed out and there are no large chunks.
6. In a bowl, combine tofu with the eggs, soy sauce and vinegar (add more soy sauce and vinegar to taste if needed).
7. Slice soft mozzarella or grate regular. Crumble goat cheese.
8. Put some sauce in bottom of an 8 x 12 inch baking dish. Place 3 rice noodles across bottom.
9. Add 1/2 the tofu mix. Top with 1/2 of each cheese then spoon 1/2 sauce on top of everything.
10. Repeat layers. You may withhold the goat cheese for sprinkling on top of sauce if desired.
11. Bake while covered at 375 degrees Fahrenheit for 35 minutes.
12. Uncover and bake for 10 additional minutes.
13. Let stand 10 minutes before cutting.

Easy Veggie Trio

Ingredients

1 large onion, chopped
Oil (Preferably something that tolerates hat well such as grape seed or coconut oils)
One package frozen black-eyed peas (16 ounces)
One bunch of fresh kale salt

1 cup water

Preparation

1. In a very large pot, cook the onion in the oil until it is translucent.
2. Add 1 cup water and the black-eyed peas, and then bring to a boil.
3. Once boiling, reduce heat and cook 20 minutes.
4. Pull the leaves off the kale stems and tear them into bite sized pieces.
5. Add the kale leaves to the pot, and stir occasionally until the kale is wilted.
6. Cover and cook until the kale is tender.
7. Add salt to taste.

Conclusion

Thank you again for downloading this book!

I hope this book was able to help you by casting some light on the importance of considering your blood type and its influence over your whole body – along with the necessity to develop an individualized diet pattern according to your blood group. In this decisive world, it's very easy to be fooled by overstated commercials urging you to take this magic pill, eat unlimited and still lose weight. However, you must think twice before you buy these magic solution products. Your body and mind deserve the best care they can get, and taking proper care of them requires persistence in pursuing a life style and a special diet plan that promote health and wellbeing. A blood type diet can guide you to move in the right direction towards that goal. This diet combines three virtues: an individualized diet, an individualized exercise regimen and lifestyle changes. Because of this, you will have your special individual issues addressed, and your special individual needs met, and you will be well on your way of taking care of your body in all its uniqueness.

You will need to build up momentum, and then follow these guidelines consistently for a long period of time. If you have any question regarding the diet plan or any other relevant questions, you may like to visit Dr. James D'Adamo 's website and get your questions answered there. You will be happy to know that about 71-78% people who have adopted a blood type diet have reported positive results.

Finally, if you enjoyed this book, please take the time to share your thoughts and post a review on Amazon. It'd be greatly appreciated!

Thank you and good luck!

Made in United States
Orlando, FL
01 May 2025